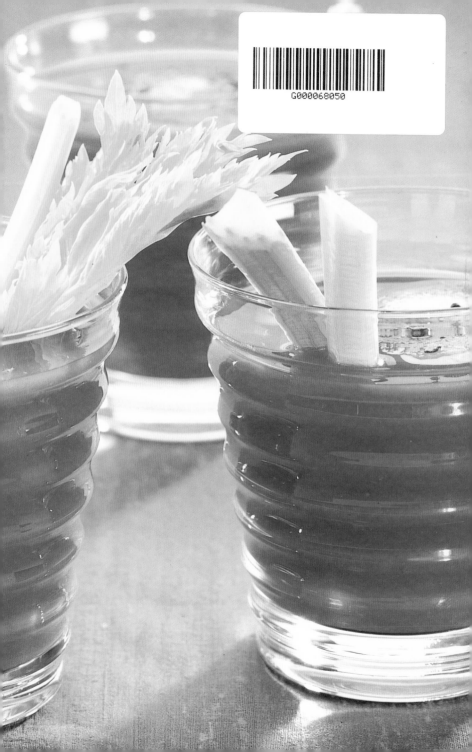

50 WAYS TO CURE A
HANGOVER

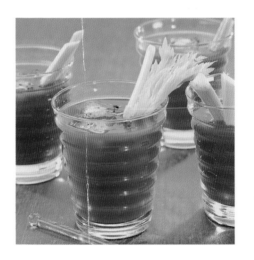

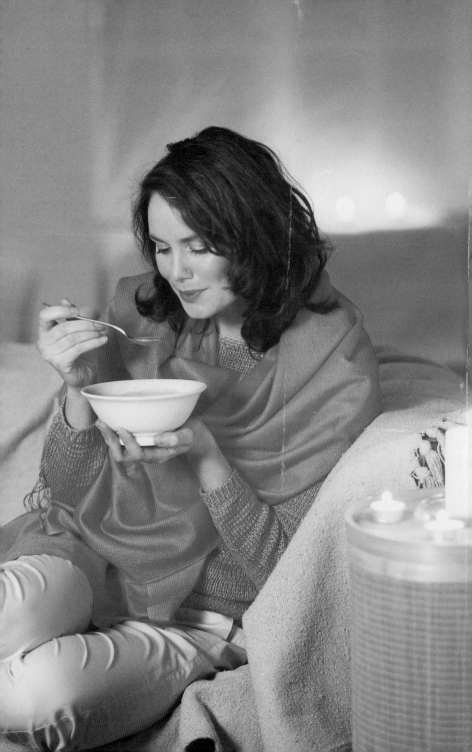

50 WAYS TO CURE A

HANGOVER

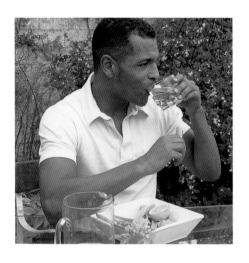

Natural remedies and therapies
shown in 70 photographs

Raje Airey

LORENZ BOOKS

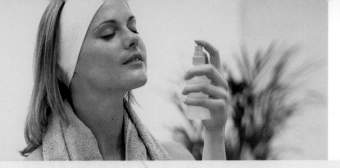

contents

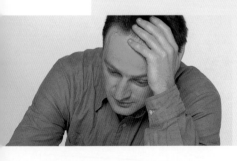

50 natural ways to...

relieve a hangover

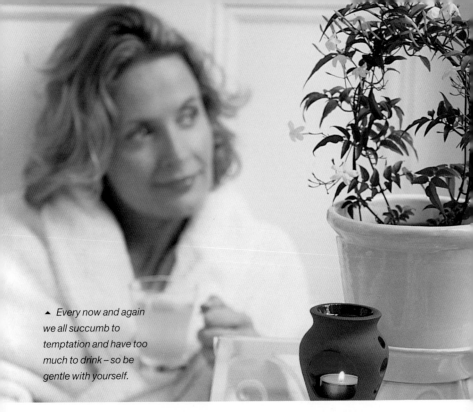

▲ *Every now and again we all succumb to temptation and have too much to drink – so be gentle with yourself.*

introduction

Dog breath, a throbbing head, churning stomach and a mouth like the inside of a birdcage. If these nasty symptoms sound horribly familiar then there is every chance that you are one of the countless millions of people who knows exactly what it feels like to suffer from a hangover. According to the dictionary, a hangover may be defined as the unpleasant effects resulting from excessive alcohol consumption. It literally means a remnant from the past (a hang-over) – or in other words, it is the morning after the night before.

So why exactly do you feel quite so ghastly? Put simply, alcohol is a drug with fairly brutal side effects. When consumed in moderate amounts, your body can produce enough enzymes to metabolize the toxins from the alcohol and you don't notice any adverse reactions. But when your level of alcohol consumption exceeds your body's ability to cope, you have all the nasty symptoms of a classic hangover. These include headaches, nausea, diarrhoea, dehydration and dizziness, together with irritability, fatigue and general aches and pains. They are the telltale signs that your body is struggling to deal with toxic overload and are a mild and temporary version of what drug addicts suffer when they experience withdrawal symptoms. A hangover is nature's way of telling you that you have been overdoing it.

congenial congeners

The excess toxins in your system seem to come from two sources. Some are present in the alcoholic drink itself, while others get created as a metabolic by-product of the liver. During the fermentation process of certain fruits or grains, the chemical compound ethanol (alcohol) is produced and this is what is responsible for a drink's intoxicating effect. At the same time, toxic by-products of the fermentation process are also created. Known as 'congeners', these chemical impurities contribute to each drink's characteristic taste, colour and aroma, and are what the liver must process. Hence it is a good idea to avoid mixing your drinks as this means the body has to work even harder in its clean-up operations. As a rule, clear wines and spirits such as vodka, gin or white wine contain fewer congeners than dark, full-bodied alcoholic drinks such as red wine, brandy or bourbon. Although congeners do not cause drunkenness, they do seem to contribute to how ill you feel afterwards. This may help to explain why the effect of drinking lighter coloured liquors seems to be slightly less devastating than drinking dark ones, an idea supported by medical research.

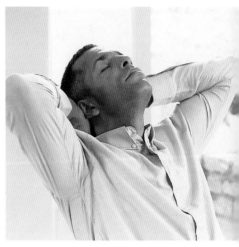

▲ The next day it can be hard to recall what was so wonderful about the night before.

feeling unwell

When the alcohol enters your bloodstream, your liver starts to produce an enzyme called 'alcohol dehydrogenase' (ADH) to break it down. Habitual drinkers have built up higher levels of ADH, which helps to explain their increased tolerance to alcohol. There is also some research to suggest that men tend to produce more of this enzyme than women and are thus able to 'hold' their drink better. As the liver gets to work, the enzymes also produce acetaldehyde, a highly toxic substance that can make you feel very unwell.

As alcohol is a diuretic, your kidneys are geared into action to pass more water than usual. It is also the body's way of trying to eliminate toxins as speedily as possible. If you do not compensate with extra liquid (non-alcoholic of course), then this impacts on the rest of the body as

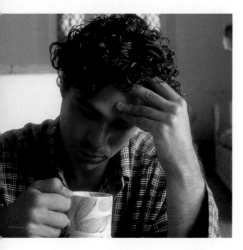

◀ *A thumping headache is a common hangover symptom. This is partly the result of being dehydrated.*

you know drinking too much is bad for you, and however many times you've sworn 'never again', there's every chance that sooner or later you're going to overdo it and once more seek solace in your favourite hangover remedy.

natural treatments
Before turning to the painkillers and pumping more drugs into your system, there are ways of treating a hangover that can support your body's natural processes rather than simply obliterating the pain. Whether you are suffering a crashing headache, a queasy tummy, or general debility, this book is packed with a variety of drug-free treatments to help alleviate some of the symptoms of a hangover. It is hoped that you will find the suggestions fun as well as useful and discover a variety of different treatments that will work for you.

whatever fluid is available is redistributed, leading to dehydration – with even your brain becoming dry and 'pickled'. This loss of body fluids is considered to be one of the major causes of hangover symptoms and, of course, is exacerbated by vomiting and diarrhoea. Although it may feel awful, vomiting and/or diarrhoea is actually a healthy response since it is the body's way of throwing out the poisons that are flooding your system.

never say never again
Excess drinking on a regular basis puts a great strain on your body. It is an addictive, expensive habit that has many unpleasant and harmful side effects. Too much alcohol depletes the body of essential vitamins and minerals and adversely affects blood sugar levels. High blood pressure, liver damage, digestive disorders, impaired mental functioning, as well as unhealthy, tired-looking skin are just some of the consequences of long-term alcohol abuse. Yet although

GOLDEN RULES
Before going out on the town, remember the following and you may save yourself an awful hangover experience.
- never drink on an empty stomach.
- eat absorbent 'bulky' foods rather than crisps, sticks of celery or nuts.
- don't mix your drinks.
- alternate each alcoholic drink with a non-alcoholic one.

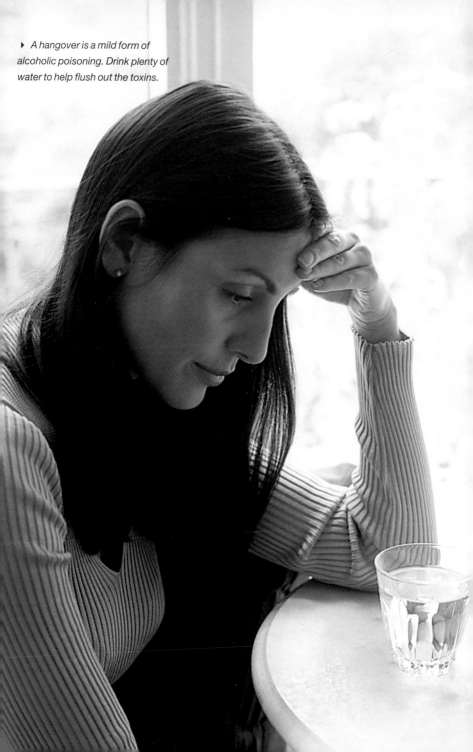

▶ *A hangover is a mild form of alcoholic poisoning. Drink plenty of water to help flush out the toxins.*

hangover treatments

The quest for the perfect hangover cure is rather like the search for the Holy Grail. It has enduring fascination yet somehow remains tantalizingly out of reach. After centuries of ingenious suggestions it is probably fairly safe to conclude that there is no single perfect cure for a hangover – other than letting nature take its course. But there are steps you can take to help nature do its work and support a speedy recovery.

The pages that follow present 50 tried and tested safe and natural treatments. Some of these are aimed at quick-fix solutions while others are targeted at improving your body's defences and strengthening resistance to hangover symptoms. They are drawn from a variety of approaches to natural healthcare and include holistic therapies such as homeopathy, reflexology, aromatherapy and colour healing, as well as diet and nutrition where a wide variety of healing foods and drinks as well as herbs and vitamins are included.

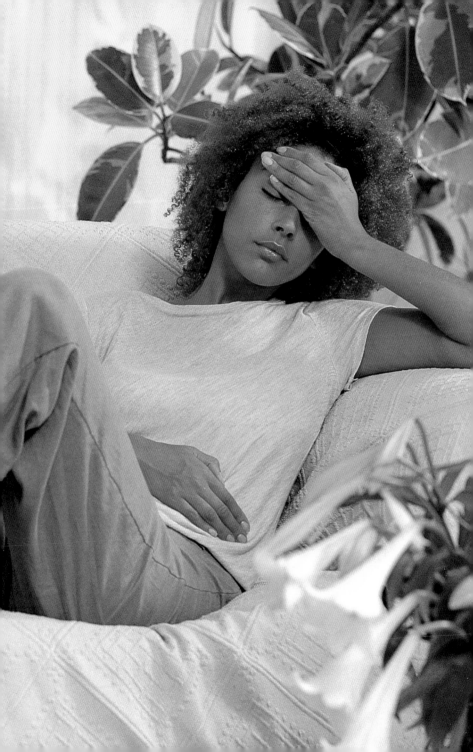

1

strengthening echinacea

Fairly new in Western herbalism, echinacea is a traditional Native American medicine. The plant's healing powers were allegedly discovered as an antidote to snakebites.

In the 1950s Ben Black Elk, a Sioux from South Dakota, gave a parting gift to the visiting Swiss 'nature' doctor Alfred Vogel. This gift was a handful of seeds from the coneflower (*Echinacea purpurea*) plant, the most powerful remedy Black Elk knew. Nowadays, echinacea is widely cultivated for its amazing healing properties. Although the plant has a particularly strong affinity with the respiratory tract, it is also a powerful blood cleanser and immunity booster.

building defences

Echinacea may not ease your hangover headache, but taken regularly it will help build and strengthen your immune system, keep your system clean and assist a speedy recovery when you do get sick – whether from illness or the effects of alcohol poisoning. During the party season when late nights, too much booze and poor eating habits are guaranteed to take their toll, using echinacea will help build your body's defences so you can party until you drop.

Echinacea is prepared as a herbal remedy from the plant's roots and

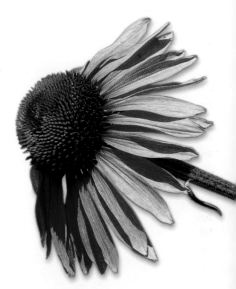

▲ *Echinacea is a powerful immunity booster. Take it regularly as a preventative measure to strengthen your system.*

leaves, although the best remedies are allegedly those that are made using the entire plant. It is available in tincture or tablet form from good health stores and pharmacies. As a preventative measure, you could take 2.5ml (½ tsp) tincture in a little water or juice once a day, or one 500mg capsule twice a day.

2 ginseng boost

In Chinese medicine, ginseng is the number one tonic and healer. For centuries in the East, top grade roots have been valued more highly than gold and imbued with almost magical properties.

In parts of Asia, ginseng plants up to 200 years old can still be found. It is believed that those lucky enough to acquire such plants can live to a ripe old age, as ginseng is said to increase longevity. Ginseng has a strengthening effect on the nervous system and improves tolerance to stress. It also aids recovery from illness, fights fatigue and boosts alertness. Although there are many varieties of ginseng, the Korean variety (*panax ginseng*) is believed to be the most powerful. Siberian ginseng (*eleutherococcus*) has a similar action and is particularly helpful for combating fatigue.

body balancer

Ginseng is a useful hangover remedy because it works to bring the body back into balance. It contains vitamins, minerals and amino acids, and helps to balance blood sugar levels in the body. Ginseng helps to protect and strengthen the liver against toxic overload. It is also a powerful immune system booster and helps combat the effects of stress. All very important if you want to avoid feeling lousy.

Although it is possible to make ginseng tea by boiling up the powdered root, most people find it more convenient to take regular supplements in tablet form, widely available in good health stores and pharmacies. Take up to two 600mg tablets daily, or as directed.

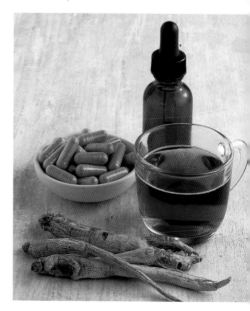

▸ *Ginseng root may be boiled up in a little water to make a tea or else it is available as a tincture or as capsules.*

3

milk thistle detox

In herbal medicine, milk thistle has a long tradition of use. It is the herbal remedy most commonly used for healing and protecting the liver and its many metabolic activities.

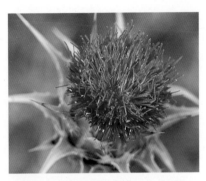

▲ Milk thistle is a powerful liver protector.

Native to the Mediterranean regions, this silvery-edged thorny leaved plant thrives in humid, salty sea air and stony soil where it can grow up to 2m (6ft) high. Silymarin, the active component of milk thistle (*Silybum marianum*), is found in the plant's seeds and it is this substance that is so effective in protecting the liver.

liver reviver

Studies have shown that silymarin can prevent severe liver damage after ingesting highly toxic compounds, while it has also been used successfully to treat hepatitis and liver cirrhosis. Milk thistle can help to regenerate a damaged liver and stimulate the production of healthy new cells; it also has a cleansing and purifying effect and encourages the liver to work more efficiently.

It is these therapeutic actions that make milk thistle such a valuable hangover remedy, as it is the liver that has to cope with all the nasty effects caused by alcoholic excess. When you have a busy social time ahead, try taking a four-week preventative course. A suggested dose would be one 500mg capsule three times a day. Or take one 500mg capsule three times a day as a first-aid measure when you have a hangover. Milk thistle is also available in tincture form.

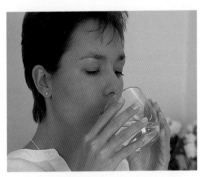

▲ A milk thistle capsule taken with a glass of water should help a hangover.

4 cleansing artichokes

Most of us are familiar with globe artichokes as a rather exotic looking vegetable. Yet this tasty plant also has an important reputation in herbal medicine for treating liver disorders.

Like milk thistle, the artichoke (*Cynara scolymus*) plant is native to the Mediterranean region. Similarly, it is also recognized as a valuable liver tonic. The green parts of the plant contain the compound cynaropicrin, which is what gives the vegetable its characteristic aroma and bitter taste. This bitterness stimulates liver and gall-bladder function, making the artichoke useful for the treatment of gall-bladder problems and digestive disorders. The plant's leaves also contain cynarin, another valuable substance that acts on the liver in a similar way to silymarin, found in milk thistle. In addition, artichokes are rich in antioxidants.

liver cleanser

Taking artichoke will help protect your liver against toxins and minimize the damage caused by drinking alcohol. It will also encourage a speedier clean-up operation. Like most herbal remedies, the plant is commercially available in tincture or capsule form, which makes it easy to use. To treat a hangover, take one 500mg capsule three times a day. Alternatively try a short course to help your liver detox, taking one 500mg capsule three times a day for four weeks. Eating the fresh vegetable is also helpful.

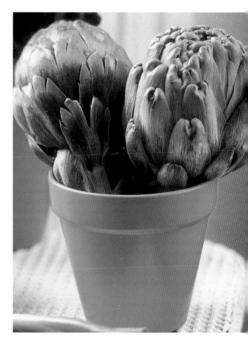

▸ *Artichokes have a distinctive, bitter taste that stimulates liver function. The herbal remedy is a good detoxifier.*

5

soothing slippery elm

Best known as a herb for treating stomach complaints, slippery elm's soothing action is wonderful for an overwrought digestive system. It should help to settle your upset stomach.

The slippery elm (*Ulmus rubra*) tree is native to Canada and the United States. It is the tree's inner bark that is used in herbal medicine. The trees must be at least ten years old and during the spring, their bark is collected, dried and then powdered. Slippery elm bark contains a viscous solution (mucilage) which gives rise to its 'slippery' taste and texture – and also the tree's name. This mucilage has a soothing action in the gut, reducing inflammation and calming spasms, making it a useful herbal remedy for a wide range of digestive disorders, including acid indigestion, diarrhoea and gastroenteritis.

speedy stomach settler

Slippery elm is available in good health stores and pharmacies and is usually sold in either powder, capsule or tablet form. For instant relief from an upset stomach, make yourself a nourishing – if slimy – drink from the powder. Mix a little powder to a paste with cold water and then top up with hot water, using a ratio of 1 part powder to 8 parts water, or follow the instructions on the jar. If you prefer, substitute the hot water with hot milk, particularly if it's last thing at night, as this may help you sleep. If you feel too sick to stomach it, then take your slippery elm in tablet or capsule form and this should help settle your heaving insides. A 400mg dose should be sufficient, followed by two 200mg doses at three-hourly intervals if needed.

◄ *Slippery elm is not to everyone's taste but it is a good stomach soother.*

6 calming ginger

Fiery ginger has been used as a culinary spice and medicine since antiquity. It is one of the best natural remedies for nausea and vomiting and a tonic for the digestive system.

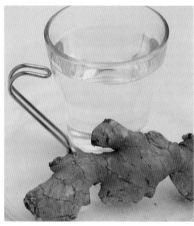

▲ *A glass of fresh ginger tea will help to settle your stomach and alleviate nausea.*

The ginger (*Zingiber officinale*) plant is cultivated throughout the tropics. Its thick, tuberous root (rhizome) is valuable, both as a food and as a medicine. The rhizome contains high levels of the plant's warming and stimulating oil. It is these invigorating properties that make ginger such a valuable medicine.

sickness suppressor
Ginger is probably best known as an antidote to nausea and vomiting, whether this is caused by motion sickness, morning sickness in pregnancy, or sickness caused by over-indulgence. There is plenty of evidence to back up ginger's effectiveness in this area: medical trials in hospitals for instance have found ginger to be more effective than conventional medicines at relieving post-operative nausea. Ginger helps to settle the stomach and ease abdominal pain, distension and flatulent indigestion as well as relaxing muscular spasm. It is also a powerful antioxidant, inhibiting free radicals in the body and stimulating the speedy removal of toxins. It is to all these properties that ginger owes its reputation as a good hangover cure.

There are a variety of ways to take ginger. The crystallized root can be chewed as a sweet, the powdered root can be taken in capsule form, or the fresh root may be boiled to make a drink. Ginger is also available in tincture form. Add 3–4 drops to a glass of water and sip at intervals. (Note: the tincture should not be confused with ginger essential oil, which is not suitable for ingestion.)

7 evening primrose oil

One of nature's most valuable plants, evening primrose is best known for its oil. This contains many nourishing properties and is said to counter the effects of alcoholic poisoning.

The fragrant yellow flowers of the evening primrose plant (*Oenothera biennis*) open at dusk, attracting the night-flying insects that pollinate them. The plant was known to the Ancient Greeks, and the flower's generic name is derived from two Greek words: 'oinos' meaning wine, and 'thera' meaning hunt. This refers to the plant's reputation to stimulate a desire for wine and/or to dispel the effects of over-indulgence. You can only judge for yourself how far this is true, but a great deal of research has been made into the medicinal effects of evening primrose oil, which is derived from the plant's seeds.

system replenisher

Evening primrose oil is an excellent source of Omega 6 fatty acids, which are vital for the healthy functioning of the immune, nervous and hormonal systems. Evening primrose oil also contains gamma linolenic acid (GLA), a precursor of prostaglandin E1 – a mood enhancer. Unfortunately alcoholic binges upset the healthy functioning of the body's systems and this enhancer can be destroyed.

Taking evening primrose oil can help to realign metabolic disturbances after drinking. Studies have also shown that it can help with alcohol withdrawal symptoms and alcoholic depression, as well as helping the liver to regenerate. The most convenient way of taking evening primrose oil is in capsules, widely available in health stores and pharmacies. For a hangover take 3-5 1000mg capsules. Evening primrose is sometimes blended with starflower oil, which works in a similar way.

▲ *Evening primrose oil can help with the symptoms of alcohol withdrawal.*

8

vitamin C

Drinking alcohol, along with smoking and stress, rapidly uses up vitamin C. This vitamin plays an essential role in maintaining a healthy immune system.

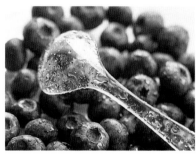

▲ Fresh blueberries are a rich and natural source of vitamin C.

Vitamin C is one of the most important vitamins needed to sustain life, yet studies show that surprisingly large numbers of people are vitamin C deficient.

Also known as ascorbic acid, vitamin C is water-soluble and any excess is excreted when you urinate. As your body is unable to store or produce this vitamin, it relies on you having an adequate daily intake.

vitamin C sources
Some of the best natural sources include rosehips, blackcurrants, citrus fruits, berries and broccoli, although it is also found in all other fresh fruit and vegetables. In addition, many people like to supplement their daily intake with vitamin pills or powders.

Normally, vitamin C is excreted in two to three hours, but because alcohol is a diuretic, elimination is faster and your body's need for vitamin C dramatically increases. If you are a smoker, the situation is compounded as it is estimated that each cigarette destroys 25mg of vitamin C. To help redress the balance, a therapeutic dose of 1000mg should help you on the way to recovery. This dose can be repeated every two to three hours as needed. If you are taking ginseng, leave a three-hour gap before or after taking vitamin C.

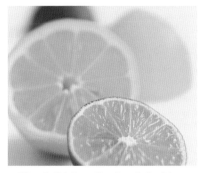

▲ Vitamin C is found in citrus fruits. It is an immunity booster and antioxidant.

9

B-complex vitamins

The B vitamins are synergistic, which means they work best when taken together as a B-complex. It is vitamin B1, however, that offers most protection against alcoholic excess.

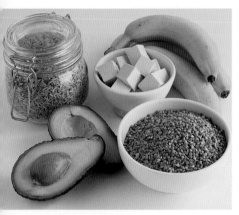

▲ *Avocados, bananas, tofu, brown rice and most wholegrains are all high in B vitamins.*

There are more than ten members of the vitamin B group and they play an essential role in more than 60 metabolic reactions. They are particularly involved in energy production and in the manufacture of red blood cells but are probably most well known for their effect on the nervous system.

vitamin B sources

As a rule, B vitamins are found more abundantly in vegetables rather than fruit, although avocados and bananas are high in B vitamins. Other good natural sources include wheat bran, yeast, fish, liver, eggs, milk and cheese.

Known as the 'feel good' vitamin, B1 (thiamine) has a beneficial effect on mood and general wellbeing, helping you feel calm, clear-headed and energetic. Low levels of thiamine are associated with lack of self-confidence and depression. Caffeine, alcohol, stress and smoking are all enemies of B1 and it may come as little surprise to find that B1 deficiency is very common. However, of all the B vitamins, it is B1 that seems to offer the most protection against a hangover and is even reputed to decrease your taste for alcohol. It is found in all plant and animal foods, but especially rich sources are brown rice, wholegrains, seafood and legumes.

To help prevent a hangover, take one high-strength B-complex tablet before drinking, one during drinking and one before you go to bed. To ease the symptoms of a hangover, take a high-strength B-complex together with a multi-vitamin and mineral tablet and repeat six hours later.

10 water, water, water

Dehydration is one of the main reasons for feeling hung over. While you are enjoying alcoholic beverages your body is actually losing fluids. Drinking water is a top cure.

The importance of drinking water cannot be stressed enough. Your body is largely made up of this vital, life-giving element and it covers more than two-thirds of the earth's surface. It is not for nothing that it is called the elixir of life.

keep topping up
To stop yourself feeling like death the morning after, make sure you drink plenty of water before you go out drinking, plenty more while you are indulging, a large glass of the stuff before you go to bed, and another large glass when you wake up. In any case health experts recommend that you should be drinking at least 1.5 litres/2½ pints/6¼ cups a day to keep you in tip-top condition – and that is before a drop of alcohol has passed your lips.

Drinking plenty of water before, during and after a drinking session will help your body in two main ways. Alcohol is a diuretic and dehydrates your body fairly dramatically. Drinking plenty of water helps to hydrate your body in preparation for the huge fluid loss caused by the booze. Secondly, it will help flush out the evil toxins that are making you feel so dreadful. Don't worry if you need to urinate more than normal – it's a small price to pay given the circumstances.

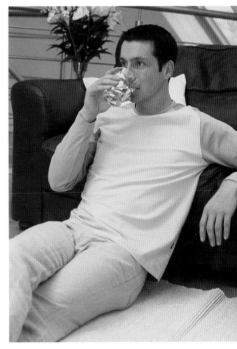

▲ Drinking plenty of water is one of the easiest ways to treat a hangover.

11 spicy orange zinger

When you feel like crawling under a stone to die, zing is probably the last thing on your mind. Yet this spicy fruit cocktail can soon change that.

Fresh fruit juices can send a hangover on its way. Like water, juices help to flush your system of toxins and rehydrate your body, which will hopefully quieten that loud, thumping headache and get rid of that awful giddy feeling.

ancient remedy

The following drink combines fresh fruit juices with spices and is based on a traditional Ayurvedic remedy. Originating in India, Ayurveda is one

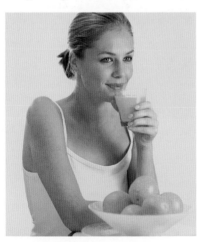

▲ *Freshly squeezed orange, lime and cumin is an Ayurvedic hangover remedy.*

of the oldest healthcare systems in the world and makes great use of nutritious foods and drinks in its treatments. Spices in particular are very important, as it is not just their taste that counts, but each has unique healing properties. To make enough for one serving, you will need the juice of 2-3 freshly squeezed large oranges, plus 10ml/2 tsp fresh lime juice and a pinch of cumin. Give the ingredients a good stir to mix well and serve immediately as fresh juices lose their potency if they are left standing around for too long.

The drink should not only taste delightful to your jaded taste buds but it is also packed with nutrients. Both oranges and limes of course are high in vitamin C and will give your immune system a much-needed boost. In Ayurvedic medicine, cumin is seen to have a cooling effect on the body and is therefore helpful in disorders associated with excess heat. After over-indulging, acid indigestion and wind are just some of the signs of an inflamed digestive system. So drink up and restore your body to balance as quickly and painlessly as possible.

12 virgin bloody mary

The reason you feel so awful is because your body is going through mild withdrawal symptoms from an alcohol overdose. Try this if you feel tempted by a curative top-up.

A Bloody Mary is a vodka and tomato juice cocktail and is probably one of the most infamous hangover cures of all. It is based on the 'hair of the dog' principle, which argues that since your hangover is caused by withdrawal symptoms, if you give yourself a top-up with more alcohol, your ghastly symptoms will subside and you will soon feel better. Ironically there is some truth in this. The effects, however, are only temporary and eventually you will have to sober up and face the loud, discordant music going on inside your skull. In any case you probably know deep down that it's not really a good idea to succumb to temptation. It will only mask your symptoms temporarily and if it became a habit, it could lead to alcohol abuse and a serious drinking problem.

healthy 'hair of the dog'
If all this sounds boringly sensible, then trick yourself with the next best thing. This Virgin Bloody Mary looks and almost tastes the same as the genuine article but it won't cause you any harm. In fact it is more than likely

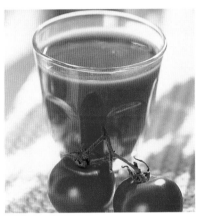

▲ Raw tomatoes contain over 90 per cent water and are said to be good for reducing liver inflammation.

to do you some good – tomatoes are alkali forming, and help to reduce stomach acidity. To make one serving you will need 300ml/½ pint/1¼ cups fresh or bottled tomato juice, juice of ½ lemon, Tabasco sauce, Worcestershire sauce, salt and pepper. Mix the tomato and lemon juice together and season to suit your taste with the rest of the ingredients. Finally, add a handful of ice for that wonderful clinking sound, put your feet up and sip through a long straw.

13

blackcurrant & cranberry breeze

When you're out on a drinking spree, your kidneys are working extra hard to flush the fluids from your system. Why not give them a helping hand with this tasty tonic?

Blackcurrants and cranberries each deserve their well-earned reputation as 'super foods'. Both fruits have a high vitamin C content and are rich in nutrients and healing properties. This makes their juice a wonderful tonic for a body under stress – an apt description for your poor hung-over system.

Blackcurrants have a blood cleansing and purifying action, while a compound in their purple-black skin is a powerful anti-inflammatory.

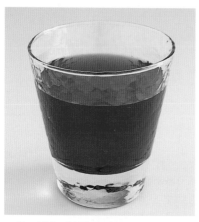

▲ Combining blackcurrant and cranberry juice makes a tasty, healing tonic which is especially beneficial for your kidneys.

This is what makes blackcurrants such a good sore throat remedy, but the same soothing properties can be put to good use to ease acid indigestion, relax intestinal spasms and stem diarrhoea. Cranberries on the other hand, with their antibacterial and strengthening properties, have a specific affinity with the kidneys and urinary tract. They have a tart, bitter taste and so work well when mixed with sweeter fruits like blackcurrants.

refresher juice

To make enough for one serving you will need 75g/3oz blackcurrants and 150g/5oz cranberries. You will also need a juicing machine. Remove the stalks from the blackcurrants and rinse the currants and the cranberries. Do not chop or peel. Put the fruit through the juicer and add a little honey to taste. If fresh fruits are not available, or you simply can't be bothered, then use ready-made juices instead. Cranberry is available in most supermarkets, while blackcurrant is sold in all good health stores. Make sure it is blackcurrant juice rather than a cordial.

14 banana smoothie

Potassium is one of the body's most important minerals and is seriously depleted through alcoholic excess. Bananas are one of the best sources of potassium.

Potassium is crucial for body functioning. It maintains the water balance within your body's cells and stabilizes their internal structure. It also plays a central role in energy production and helps to conduct nerve impulses through the body. When your body loses fluids, whether through sweating, vomiting, diarrhoea, or from diuretics, then potassium is leached away. Symptoms of potassium deficiency include muscular weakness, muscle pains and overwhelming fatigue, which are all common hangover symptoms.

energy boosting bananas
Bananas are packed with potassium and are an instant energy food. They also contain zinc, iron, and vitamins C and B6. Natural antacids, bananas can also restore an angry digestive system to normal functioning. For maximum benefit, bananas should be eaten ripe; they are less effective when they are still green around the tips. Avoid bruised or greyish bananas, but opt for plump fruit with a good colour.

For an instant energy-boosting drink that will also soothe your weary system this banana smoothie should do the trick. This delicious thick and fruity drink is mixed with yogurt and/or milk.

To make enough for one serving you will need 1 good-sized ripe banana, 120ml/4fl oz/½ cup skimmed milk and 50ml/2fl oz/¼ cup natural live yogurt. Peel the banana and put all the ingredients into a blender and blend until smooth. Add more milk if you like a runnier consistency and serve chilled or on ice.

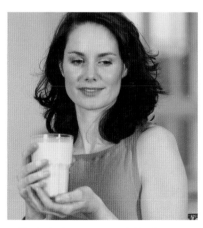

▲ *For instant energy, a nourishing banana smoothie will soon put the bounce back in your step.*

15 green energy

Fresh juices have remarkable cleansing and restorative powers. Green veggie juices in particular are great for detoxing the body's systems and strengthening the liver.

A detox programme is the classical treatment for weaning addicts off alcohol and drugs. Although no one is suggesting that you are alcohol dependent, a detox remains one of the best natural treatments for a hangover. For a simple detox, drinking fresh vegetable juice is one of the simplest and most effective cures. Vegetable juices have a much milder action in the body than fruit juices and are also excellent restoratives and should soon put you back on your feet.

Chlorophyll is the 'green blood' of plants that enables them to harvest the sun's life-giving energy. It has potent cleansing properties and is what makes green vegetables so helpful in a detox. As a rule, the darker green the vegetable, the more potent its potential detoxing and curative powers. Dark green vegetables are also rich in B vitamins and minerals.

detox veggie juice

This 'green energy' juice is made from spinach and celery, although you could substitute watercress, curly kale or cabbage for the spinach if you prefer. Celery is included for its high water content and its toning effect on the kidneys. According to traditional herbal medicine it also calms the nerves. To make enough for one serving you will need 2 sticks of celery and a large handful of spinach leaves. Wash the veggies and put them in a juice extractor. If you wish, you could mix with a little fresh carrot juice for flavour. Drink up immediately, as the juice will lose its potency if it is left standing around.

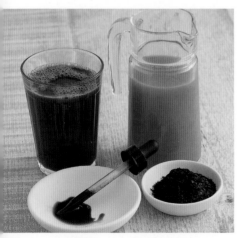

▲ Dark green vegetable juices are potent detoxifiers and energy boosters.

16

prairie oyster

The desire for a hangover cure has led to many strange experimental remedies. Raw eels, soused herrings and raw eggs have all been popular. A prairie oyster is a type of egg nog.

In the Middle Ages, hangover sufferers swore by a mixture that included raw eel, while in Holland a whole soused herring slipped down the back of the throat is meant to work wonders. It's difficult to know on what basis some of these cures are founded, suffice to say that if you can swallow it down without throwing it up then you must be on the way to a speedy recovery – or else you're still too drunk to notice!

eggy hangover cure

A prairie oyster is based on the 'hair of the dog that bit me' premise and uses a vodka or brandy base. It is equally effective without the alcohol as it is the raw egg that does the trick. Maybe this is because eggs contain cysteine, which is said to clean up destructive chemicals that build up in the liver while metabolizing excess alcohol.

To make a prairie oyster mix 25ml/ 1½ tbsp apple cider vinegar, 25ml/ 1½ tbsp Worcestershire sauce, 5ml/ 1 tsp tomato ketchup, 5ml/1 tsp Angostura bitters and a dash of Tabasco in a tumbler. If you really want to go for the full hair of the dog, then add 25ml/1½ tbsp of either brandy or vodka, but this is strictly optional. Finally, drop in a raw egg yolk and knock it back without breaking the yolk. Make sure that the bathroom is within striking distance!

> **CAUTIONS**
> • Children, pregnant women and the elderly should avoid eating raw eggs.
>
> • Free-range organic eggs are the safest choice when using them raw.

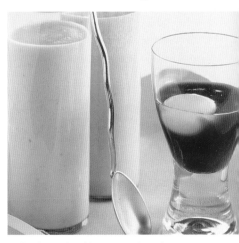

▲ *Drinks made with raw eggs have been popular hangover cures for centuries.*

17 peppermint tea

Herbal teas are excellent natural hangover remedies. Peppermint is a firm favourite as it is healing for an upset digestive system and makes a refreshing start to the day.

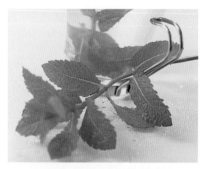

▲ Peppermint is one of the most useful and effective herbal hangover remedies.

If you feel tempted to sober up with a black coffee, think again. Coffee will dehydrate and irritate your system still further, and contrary to popular opinion, it will do nothing for your hangover – except make you feel more awake perhaps. For a therapeutic wake-up call, peppermint tea is a much better way to stimulate your groggy self into action.

reviving peppermint
Peppermint (*Mentha* **x** *piperita*) has always been valued for its stimulating, refreshing effects. Centuries ago, the Roman historian, Pliny (AD23–79) stated: 'the very smell of mint restores and revives the spirits just as its taste excites the appetite'. It is the volatile oil in the plant's leaves that creates peppermint's distinctive aroma and gives it its therapeutic powers. This essential oil should not be ingested directly, but the plant's fresh or dried leaves may be infused in hot water and made into tea.

Peppermint is a top herbal remedy for nausea and indigestion. When taken internally, it brings relief for conditions associated with pain and spasm, including stomach ache, wind, heart burn, indigestion, hiccups and vomiting. Peppermint helps to protect the gut lining from irritation and infection, and relieves griping pains during diarrhoea. It also has a cleansing and detoxing effect on the liver.

minty brew
For a refreshing peppermint tea, use 5ml/1 tsp dried peppermint leaves or 10ml/2 tsp fresh herbs per 250ml/ 8fl oz/1 cup of near-boiling water. Steep the herbs in the water for 5-10 minutes, then drain off the liquid into a cup and drink while hot. If you need a sweetener, stir in a little honey.

18

lemon, lime & ginger toddy

Like lemons, limes are high in vitamin C as well as B vitamins. Their unique citrus flavours combine with ginger in this hot toddy that will ease a horrible hangover.

We generally think of lemons and limes as being very acidic and may conclude that they are best avoided when suffering from an upset stomach. However, the fruits' acidic properties are metabolized during digestion to produce potassium carbonate, which actually helps neutralize excess acid in the body. Furthermore, lemon juice has a protective action on the membranous lining of the digestive tract, making it useful to help prevent stomach upsets.

Both lemons and limes are also a tonic for the liver and pancreas. They have a cleansing and purifying action that helps to remove toxic wastes and impurities and restore the body to a state of homeostasis (balance). Their taste and healing properties are complemented by ginger, which in itself is an excellent remedy for nausea and stomach upsets.

comforting hot toddy

To make a lemon, lime and ginger toddy, take a 115g/4oz piece of washed fresh root ginger and slice it into 600ml/1 pint/2½ cups water. Bring the water to the boil, cover and gently simmer the root for 15-20 minutes. Meanwhile squeeze 1 medium-sized lemon and 1 lime and put the juice to one side. When the ginger has finished cooking, remove it from the heat and strain the liquid into a cup. Allow it to cool slightly before adding the citrus juices. Sweeten with honey to taste, go back to bed and sip slowly.

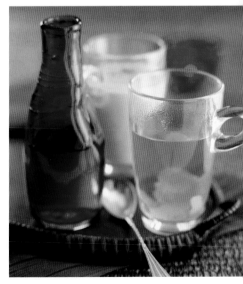

▲ A hot toddy made with lemon, lime and ginger is an excellent restorative.

19

dandelion & marshmallow brew

Although dandelion is infamous as a weed, it is important in herbal medicine because of its detoxifying, bitter properties. Combine it with marshmallow for a potent hangover drink.

Both the leaves and root of the unassuming dandelion plant (*Taraxacum officinale*) have a therapeutic action on the kidneys and liver. Dandelion's edible and bitter leaves are a powerful diuretic, but unlike most conventional diuretics that leach the body of potassium, they actually contain high levels of the mineral. This creates an ideal balance, helping the kidneys flush out toxins on the one hand, while simultaneously keeping the body's potassium levels high. Dandelion root is also a very effective detoxifying

▲ A dandelion and marshmallow herbal tea is soothing for an upset stomach.

herb. Although its main area of action is on the liver and gall-bladder, it also has a stimulating effect on the kidneys and helps the body to excrete toxins via the urine.

Known as the flower of softness, the high mucilage content of marshmallow (*althaea officinalis*) makes it useful whenever a soothing effect is needed. Marshmallow root is used primarily for stomach problems and inflammations of the digestive tract. It counters excess stomach acid and soothes an irritable bowel.

stomach settling brew

A dandelion and marshmallow brew is a fantastic detoxing hangover cure that is kind to your insides. To make a brew, add 10g/¼oz each of dried dandelion and marshmallow root to 600ml/1 pint/2½ cups water and simmer for 10 minutes. When the roots have softened add 5g/⅙oz each of dried dandelion and marshmallow leaves to the hot water, cover and leave to infuse for a further 5 minutes. If using fresh herbs, double the quantities. Strain off the liquid and drink while still warm.

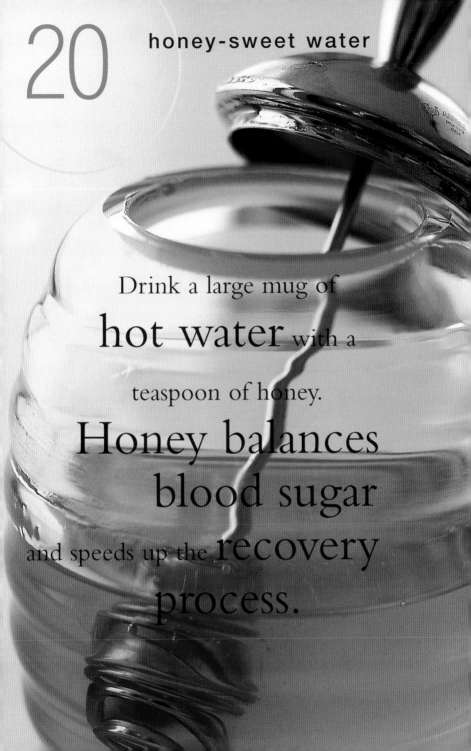

Drink a large mug of
hot water with a
teaspoon of honey.
Honey balances
blood sugar
and speeds up the recovery
process.

21 green tea

It's official – green tea is not only a refreshing drink, but it's also good for you. It has many health-giving properties and is a great way to defend yourself against a hangover.

For centuries China has praised the benefits of its native plant, and tea drinking has played an integral part in Eastern cultures – not only in China, but also in India and Japan. Today we are discovering what all the fuss was about. Research shows that regular tea drinking promotes healthy bones, skin and teeth, while its vital compounds give protection against serious diseases such as cancer and diabetes. This is particularly true for green tea, which is packed with health-giving flavonoids as well as vitamins and minerals. Its caffeine content is also negligible.

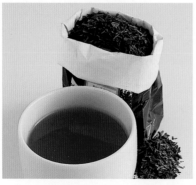

▲ Green tea is packed with goodness and will help your body return to health.

powerful properties

Green tea is a potent antioxidant with antibacterial and anti-inflammatory properties. It is also an immunity booster and helps keep you fighting fit so that your body is better able to process harmful substances. It has a cooling, cleansing action on your body and drinking it after you've over-indulged will help your system deal with the toxic overload while soothing any gastric upsets. It also has a head-clearing effect and will help you focus on the day ahead.

There are many varieties of green tea to choose from. Take your pick from Chinese green jasmine, Japanese bancha or sencha, or a green Assam or Darjeeling from India. Look out for and experiment with new green teas as they come onto the market and decide which ones you like best. The secret of a successful green tea brew is to let the water cool off for about five minutes after boiling before pouring it onto the tea and then leaving the tea to steep for about a minute. As a preventative measure, drink two or three cups of green tea a day; for a hangover, drink as much as you can.

22 meadowsweet tisane

A tisane is a type of herbal infusion. This one is made with meadowsweet, a powerful remedy for neutralizing stomach acid. It should help ease many nasty hangover symptoms.

Meadowsweet (*Filipendula ulmaria*) is one of the best antacid remedies for indigestion and heartburn and makes a very useful hangover remedy. It relieves embarrassing and painful wind and flatulence, stems diarrhoea and soothes intestinal spasms. It also has a protective and healing action on the bowel's mucous membranes. Nicholas Culpeper, the 17th-century English herbalist, claimed that meadowsweet was of great help to those that were 'troubled with the cholic, being boiled in wine'.

pain-relieving properties

The herb has a powerful anti-inflammatory and pain-relieving action, which is attributed to the salicylate compounds found in the plant's flowering tops and leaves. When oxidized these compounds yield salicylic acid, from which acetyl-salicylic acid or aspirin can be derived. However unlike aspirin, meadowsweet also contains other constituents that protect the stomach lining while soothing painful, inflamed conditions.

To make a meadowsweet tisane, steep 25g/1oz dried herb or 40g/1½oz fresh herb in 600ml/1 pint/2½ cups of hot water, cover and infuse for about 10 minutes. This is enough to make a pot. For an extra boost, you could also try adding two to three dried clove buds to the pot. Cloves also help to reduce gas and have analgesic properties. They will give the brew a spicy lift.

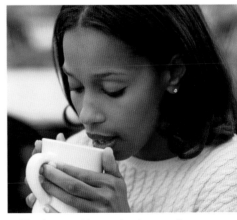

▲ *Meadowsweet has analgesic properties. Drink it in a herbal infusion.*

23 natural live yogurt

The main reason that your stomach feels as though you are sailing the ocean waves is because its delicate pH balance has been upset. Live yogurt to the rescue.

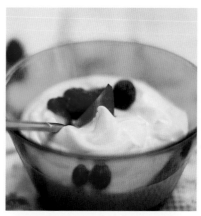

▲ *Eating live yogurt before you go out drinking can help prevent a hangover.*

Overindulgence in alcohol can cause gastritis. This is the official name for an inflammation of the stomach lining and typical symptoms include nausea, vomiting, some abdominal pain, diarrhoea and wind. Excessive alcohol consumption makes your stomach highly acidic – think green bile slopping around – which is why you feel so sick. Yogurt is an alkaline food that will help redress the balance. To work effectively, the yogurt needs to be 'live' and natural and preferably not flavoured or sweetened.

stomach soother

Eating plenty of live yogurt before you go out on a drinking spree may actually help prevent a hangover. It will line your stomach and help protect it from the acidic onslaught later on. Drinking milk has a similar effect, but live yogurt is much better because it contains natural probiotics. These are the 'friendly' bacteria that live in your intestines and are responsible for its healthy workings. It is estimated that your intestines contain about 11 trillion bacteria, 70 per cent of which should be the healthy, probiotic type. Excess alcohol, together with smoking and stress, upsets this balance.

If you didn't manage to eat yogurt before you went out, eating it after you've been drinking is the next best thing. It will soothe and cool your angry insides and help you to feel more human. If you're not keen on the taste of natural yogurt, stir in a little runny honey to sweeten. Remember that honey is also a natural antibiotic and helps the body to metabolize alcohol. It also helps alleviate a thumping headache.

24

eat your oats

Oats are a top-class 'A' grade food. They are not only rich in nutrients but are also easily digested. Because oats are an alkaline food they are soothing for an upset stomach.

It is estimated that a 90g/3½oz serving of oats contains 15g/½oz of protein. Oats are also rich in calcium, magnesium, iron and potassium and contain plenty of the B-complex vitamins. Being a wholegrain food they are high in fibre that will help to 'bulk' up the contents of your stomach (assuming there are any left) and settle things down. Traditionally oats are used in convalescence to help the body return to health. In days gone by, an oat posset made with oatmeal, water, lemon juice, sugar and spices was a standard prescription in the sickroom.

The soothing and fortifying effect of oats is not only good for your digestive tract but also your nervous system. Oats can help calm jangled nerves and lift your mood so that you feel ready to face the day with poise and grace. Oats cooked as porridge make a great start to the day. To make one serving of porridge, a 40g/1½oz serving of oats should be sufficient, unless you are very hungry.

▸ *Oats can be eaten raw in muesli or cooked and made into porridge.*

hangover muesli mix
To make a supply of homemade muesli you will need:
300g/11oz porridge oat flakes
115g/4oz malted wheat flakes
115g/4oz rye flakes
75g/3oz each of dried apricots, dates, walnuts and almonds
an airtight container

Pour the flakes into the container. Cut up the apricots and dates into small pieces, break up the nuts and add the lot to the oat base and mix well together. The muesli will keep for two to three months. You can experiment by using different fruits and nuts.

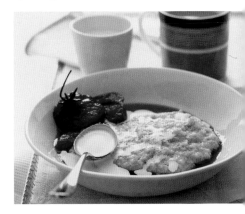

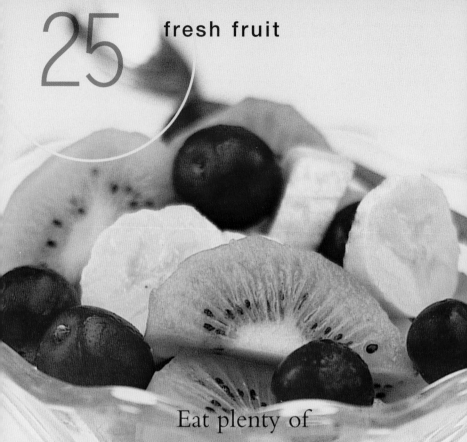

Eat plenty of
fresh fruit to cleanse and

rehydrate your system.
Apples, melons, kiwis and all the
citrus fruits are excellent.

26 sprouted seeds

For a powerhouse of goodness there is nothing to beat sprouted seeds. They contain all the plant's nutrients in a highly concentrated form and are fantastic energy boosters.

Excess alcohol really does put an enormous strain on your system. The next day it is almost impossible not to feel tired and irritable from lack of sleep, and suffer the ghastly after-effects as your body struggles to cope with toxic overload. It is no wonder that you feel like death warmed up.

hangover busting sprouts

Sprouted seeds are bursting with life. Eating them will give you energy and help your system to clean out. They are also cheap and easy to grow.

Special sprouters are available in good health stores, or alternatively you can use a large glass jar. To sprout seeds, spread a fine layer over the shelves of a sprouter or put a handful into a jar. Keep them in a light but cool spot, out of direct sunlight and water twice a day. If you are using a jar, cover the top with a mesh 'lid' made from a piece of muslin or nylon stocking. Drain off the water after watering so that the seeds are not left to lie in water. After a day or so, tiny shoots will appear. You can continue to grow the seeds for several days,

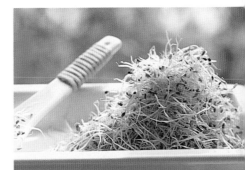

▲ Alfalfa sprouts are easy to grow and have a cleansing action on the body.

harvesting along the way. You can also buy seeds ready sprouted in supermarkets and health stores.

Some of the best seeds to sprout for a hangover are alfalfa or sunflower. Sunflower seeds strengthen your eyes' sensitivity to light and are a potent detoxifier. Alfalfa contains potassium and other minerals and has an anti-inflammatory and cleansing effect on the body. Although not a seed, mung beans are also a good choice. They are rich in minerals, B and C vitamins and are excellent for detoxification. They're also one of the easiest 'seeds' to sprout.

27 full-protein breakfast

If you can face it, a full-protein breakfast – eggs, bacon, sausages, hash browns and the like – is a tried and tested hangover cure that many hangover sufferers swear by.

Think breakfast, think big. Everyone has their favourite version of what they like in a full cooked breakfast, but the number one ingredient has to be an egg or two (or even three).

wholesome eggs
Eggs supply first-class protein, zinc and B vitamins, as well as other nutrients. They are easily digested when lightly boiled, although how people like their eggs cooked varies greatly. Eggs that are fried and 'sunny-side-up' are probably the most

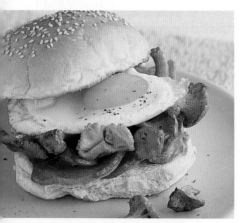

▲ A cooked breakfast with bacon and eggs is a 'kill or cure' hangover remedy.

naughty, but poached eggs will give you a yolk to dip into without the grease factor. Scrambled eggs are another good option. When buying eggs opt for free-range, as battery eggs may contain residues of factory-farming chemicals.

the full monty
Other traditional ingredients in the big breakfast include meats such as bacon, sausages and black pudding, although in some parts of the world, beefsteak is popular. The meat is usually fried or grilled. Fried potatoes such as hash browns or potato wedges are also on the menu, while fried tomatoes, mushrooms and baked beans must mean that it's good for you. The whole lot is usually accompanied by several slices of fried or toasted bread and washed down with a mug of coffee or tea.

Fans of the full-protein breakfast insist that it just 'hits the spot'. If you can keep it inside you, it will certainly keep you going for the rest of the day. If you can't face cooking and clearing up, then spoil yourself and head for the nearest diner or café.

28 super soups

For convalescents, soups are a favourite food. They are quick to prepare, packed with nutrients and help to rehydrate the body. Include soup on your day-after menu.

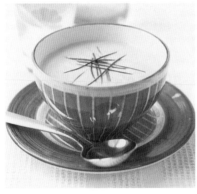

▲ *Freshly made hangover chicken soup is easy on your digestive system.*

Chicken soup is the traditional sickroom standby. This is probably because chicken has a mild antibiotic action in the body, as well as being packed with vitamins and minerals. It is also one of the easiest meats to digest and will boost energy levels.

hangover chicken soup
This hearty, appetizing soup contains barley, which consists of plenty of B-complex vitamins, potassium and other minerals. It also has a soothing action on the stomach, intestines and urinary tract.

1 large onion
15ml/1 tbsp olive oil
1 large carrot
4 sticks celery
1 litre/1¾ pints/4 cups
　chicken stock
1 bay leaf
ground black pepper
25ml/1½ tbsp pot barley
2-3 handfuls bite-sized, cooked
　chicken pieces, without the skin

Chop the onion and soften in the olive oil over a low heat, without letting the onion brown. Wash the rest of the vegetables and chop them into small pieces. Add them to the onion, cover and leave all the vegetables to soften for 5-10 minutes. Check the pan every now and again and give it a stir to make sure the vegetables are not sticking. Pour in the stock and add the bay leaf and enough ground black pepper to taste. Wash the barley and add to the pot, together with the chicken pieces. Bring to the boil, lower the heat and simmer for 1 hour. Check the seasoning and serve with wholemeal bread.

29

the aussie answer

The Australians have their own special recipe for dealing with the ghastly after-effects of the demon drink. This tasty omelette has a spicy kick to it that will stimulate your over-worked system.

If you can't face a big breakfast but want something substantial, this super snack could well fit the bill. It is also perfect for brunch or a light supper, so give it a try. There are several variations on the recipe, but it is basically a spicy omelette served with avocado. If it is too spicy for you, then use less chilli and omit the Tabasco.

spicy omelette

2-3 ripe but firm tomatoes
1 small green pepper (capsicum)
1 green chilli
6 eggs
salt and pepper
Tabasco sauce
120ml/4fl oz/½ cup milk
sunflower oil
1 avocado pear

Skin and chop the tomatoes. Deseed the green pepper and the chilli and chop them up into small pieces. Whisk the eggs and season with the salt and pepper and a dash of Tabasco. Add the milk and the chopped vegetables. Heat the oil in a large frying pan and pour in the egg blend and cook over a low heat. Slice the avocado while the omelette is cooking and then turn it over or brown it under the grill to cook the top. Serve while piping hot with the avocado slices as an accompaniment.

nourishing avocados

Avocado pears are almost a complete food as they contain protein and starch as well as fat. They are also rich in potassium and a good source of vitamins, while their anti-oxidizing properties make them good for countering toxicity in the body.

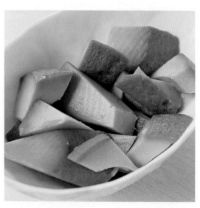

▲ Avocado pears are good for cleansing the system and help to nourish the skin.

30 homeopathic remedies

For a holistic approach to a hangover, choose a homeopathic treatment. Homeopathy considers mental and emotional 'symptoms', as well as the physical ones, and offers suitable remedies.

Homeopathic remedies are prepared from a variety of plants and mineral substances. These are then diluted many times over until no molecules of the original substance remain. It is for this reason that many people are sceptical as to how the remedies can possibly work and put it down to a placebo effect. However homeopathy has been in use for about 200 years, so you will have to decide for yourself whether homeopathy works for you.

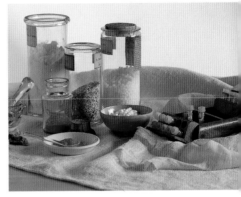

▲ Homeopathic remedies are taken as small tasteless tablets or as drops.

homeopathic hangover remedies

The practice of homeopathy is based on the principle that like-cures-like. This means that the symptoms caused by too much of a substance can also be cured by taking a small dose of it. A treatment is selected by matching your symptoms with a suitable remedy. Take the 6C potency, two tablets every hour for six doses. Coffee, peppermint, eucalyptus and other strong smells can antidote homeopathic remedies so are best avoided. Following are some of the best hangover remedies:

• **nux vomica:** the classic hangover remedy. Symptoms brought on by overindulgence in alcohol and rich food. Sufferer is irritable, impatient, and highly sensitive to light, noises and smells. Absence of thirst.

• **lycopodium:** where there is a lot of gas and heartburn. The sufferer feels better left alone but likes to know there is someone close by.

• **carbo veg:** face pale or sallow; bitter taste in mouth and burning feeling in the stomach; acid indigestion; nausea. Sluggish and irritable; better for fresh air.

• **kali bich:** hangover especially after too much beer; yellow coating on tongue; burning pains in stomach.

31 head massage

A pounding headache can be soothed away with a gentle head massage. It helps to release muscular tension and sends healing signals to the rest of the body.

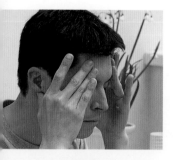

headache soother

1 Use your middle fingers to smooth out your forehead. Use a firm pressure and work from the middle, out towards the hairline. Cover the whole forehead and repeat.

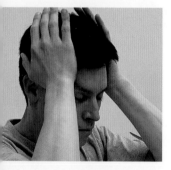

2 Position the heel of your hands over your temples and press inwards with a firm pressure. Using a circling action, work 6 times in a clockwise direction and then repeat 6 times in an anti-clockwise direction.

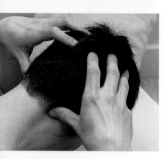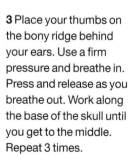

3 Place your thumbs on the bony ridge behind your ears. Use a firm pressure and breathe in. Press and release as you breathe out. Work along the base of the skull until you get to the middle. Repeat 3 times.

Massage is one of the oldest known therapies in the world. Based on the healing power of touch, it can make us feel better almost instantly. Stroking movements appear to trigger the release of endorphins, the body's natural painkillers, and induce feelings of comfort and wellbeing. Studies have also shown that massage is able to strengthen the body's immune system, lower stress levels and speed up the body's elimination of toxins.

massage technique

It is easiest to do the headache massage (left) while sitting at a table so you can support your head with your arms. If you find any particularly tight spots, these are likely to be trigger points for the headache.

32 reflexology

It may not be obvious but you can actually help your hangover by pressing certain points on your hands or feet. This special type of massage is called reflexology.

how it works

According to reflexology, the hands and feet are like a map in miniature of the whole body. When pressure is applied at certain 'reflex' points on them, it can be used to affect the corresponding areas of the body so as to stimulate natural healing. The energy booster (right) will also help strengthen the immune system.

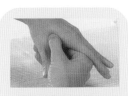

EMERGENCY FIX
There is a special pressure point between the thumb and forefinger that can help to settle an acid stomach and relieve headaches. Use your thumb to press quite hard, exhaling as you do so. Do not do if pregnant.

energy booster

1 To help strengthen the whole body, use your thumb to press firmly around the liver area. This is mid-way along the base of the right foot and is often tender.

2 Now work the digestive area, roughly the middle area of the feet. This area contains pressure points for the liver, stomach, spleen, kidneys and intestines. For sore or tender areas, hold the pressure for a little longer, while breathing out.

3 Finish by working on the upper and lower lymph systems to encourage the speedy removal of toxins. This area is on the top of each foot. Press between the toes with your finger and continue in a line down the foot.

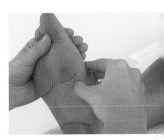

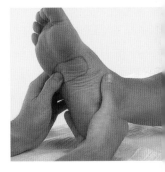

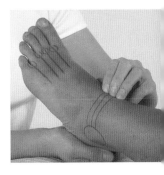

33 reiki healing

Try a gentle reiki treatment to soothe away your hangover and restore peace and calm. Reiki is a form of hands-on spiritual healing that comes from Japan.

energy therapy

In Japanese, the word 'rei-ki' means universal-life energy. When people give a reiki treatment, they 'channel' this energy. Visualizing it as a white light, they draw it in from the universe through their bodies and allow it to work through their hands.

reiki balancer

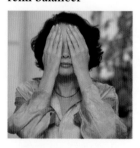

1 Place both hands over closed eyes. Imagine a white light beaming from your hands into your eyes. This should feel refreshing and will clear a heavy head.

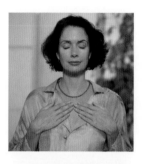

2 Place both hands on your upper chest, visualizing the white light beaming out from them. It may begin to feel warm. This position is good for lymph drainage and for clearing toxins.

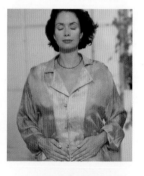

3 Move your hands to your lower abdomen, just below your navel. Continue to visualize the white light as being concentrated beneath your hands. This position transmits healing energy to your stomach and digestive system.

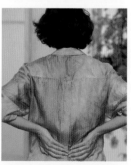

4 Finish with both of your hands resting on your lower back, just over your kidneys. Visualize the white light sending its healing energy to your kidneys and through your body.

34 crystal magic

It may sound a little far-fetched but crystals and gemstones can be used to exorcize the ill effects of the demon drink. Certain stones have special healing properties.

Crystals are used in healing to work on imbalances in the body's subtle energy system that runs through the body along invisible energy pathways (meridians) and is concentrated at energy hot spots (chakras). When we are ill, the meridians and chakras no longer work properly and our energy becomes stuck or over-stimulated. Feeling good is connected with our vital energies being balanced and flowing freely. This means that a hangover is not only affecting your physical body but is playing havoc with the subtle fine-tuning of your energy body.

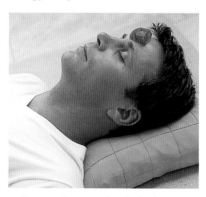

▲ To ease a hangover headache, try an amethyst crystal on your brow chakra.

To treat a hangover headache, place a stone on your brow chakra (the mid-point between the eyebrows); for an upset stomach, on the solar plexus chakra (just above the navel); to help with dehydration, on the lower abdomen chakra (just below the navel); or for low energy and general rebalancing, one on the root chakra (on the pubic bone) and one on the crown chakra (on top of your head).

hangover easing gemstones
There are many different kinds of crystals, each having particular associations and healing properties.
• **clear quartz:** for that groggy 'just let me die' feeling. Quartz strengthens, cleanses and purifies and is a good all-round rebalancer.
• **amethyst:** for a pounding headache and acid indigestion. Amethyst is calming and soothing and is said to be a cure for drunkenness.
• **garnet:** detoxifier, cleanses the blood.
• **citrine:** soothes digestive upsets; also good for liver, kidneys and colon.
• **tourmeline**: has a special affinity with the liver and kidneys; it also cleanses and strengthens.

35 flower essences

There are several flower essences that can help alleviate the symptoms of a hangover. They work primarily on a 'soul' level and help to realign the body's subtle energies when you are sick.

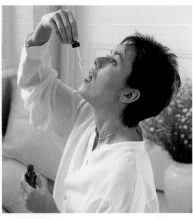

▲ Flower essence drops can be taken directly from the dropper bottle, or can be added to a glass of water or fresh juice.

Flower essences are especially useful for dealing with negative mental and emotional states. The Bach flowers are probably the most well-known system, although Australian Bush essences are also popular. Bach flowers get their name from Dr Edward Bach, an English physician, who discovered that certain plants had an effect on his mood and emotions, and that these properties could be utilized for healing. Flower remedies are prepared by infusing flower heads in water, which is believed to absorb the flower's unique vibrations. The liquid is then preserved in brandy.

hangover healers

To treat a hangover, crab apple is probably the number one remedy as it is the essence for cleansing and eliminating toxicity in mind, body and soul. Its purifying effects help to remove negativity. Hornbeam can also be helpful, particularly if you wake with a heavy head and that 'Monday morning feeling'. Hornbeam's energies have been described as a cool, refreshing shower. If you suffer hangovers a little too often, then taking chestnut bud as a preventative should help – it is the remedy for those who keep repeating the same mistakes. Take 4–6 drops, 3 times a day.

Alternatively if your symptoms are acute, then try Bach's rescue remedy or Australian Bush emergency essence. Both contain essences designed to cope with emergency situations. To treat a hangover, take 4 drops of the essence in a little water every half an hour until your symptoms subside.

36 colour therapy

The power of colour to influence mood is well known. When you're far from feeling 'in the pink', try some colour therapy to knock your hangover on the head.

Making ourselves feel better with colour is something that we do instinctively. We all know what it's like to have colour fads and how wearing a particular shade can feel just right one day but all wrong the next. Yet our choices may be based on more than a whim as different colours emit different vibrations. Remember that colour is actually light and moves in waves. Darker colours have a longer wavelength and a lower frequency, while lighter colours have a shorter wavelength and higher frequency.

The most obvious way of using colour therapeutically is to wear it as an item of clothing. Another way is to 'bathe' in coloured light by placing a special coloured gel or slide in front of a high-powered lamp, making sure that it is not touching the bulb. You can also make a colour infusion by putting coloured stones or any other colourfast item into a bowl of mineral water and leaving it to infuse for several hours, preferably in sunlight. Pour the water into a glass and drink it. Always make sure that the coloured item you are using is clean before you soak it.

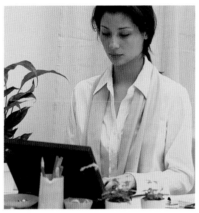

▲ When feeling under the weather, surround yourself with healing colours. Green is both detoxifying and refreshing.

colours for a hangover

You can use colour vibrations to treat many hangover symptoms. Hot reds, pinks and oranges are best avoided as they may be over-stimulating.

- **yellow:** digestive disturbances; acid indigestion, sickness, diarrhoea.
- **green:** detoxifying, cleansing.
- **blue, violet:** strengthens and protects the liver; insomnia.
- **turquoise:** immunity booster; anti-inflammatory.
- **indigo:** headaches; painkiller.

37

float away

The perfect answer! Float away without any effort, your body suspended in warm water in an environment free from external stimuli – no noise, no light. Absolute bliss.

Flotation therapy was developed in the United States during the 1970s. It involves floating in a special sound- and light-proof tank or chamber, although you can switch a light on and open the door at any time. The water is maintained at skin temperature (34.2°C/93.5°F) and contains salts and minerals so that you can float without any effort at all. The result is deep relaxation for both body and mind.

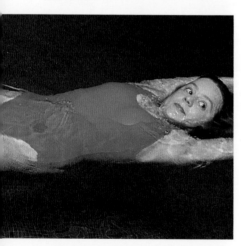

▲ Floating is profoundly relaxing and helps the body to detox. Book yourself a session at your nearest health centre.

mind and body detox

During relaxation, your brain releases endorphins, which are the body's natural painkillers. Many people find flotation to be an uplifting experience similar to meditation. It also helps the body to detox and is a great way of helping to clear a hangover. Floating is probably best tried later on in the day when any acute hangover symptoms, such as sickness and diarrhoea, have subsided. Floating is also a good immunity booster so it should help get you back on your feet in no time.

Most good health clubs have flotation facilities. There is usually a suite of private rooms containing the tank and shower facilities. The tank itself is large enough so that you can comfortably stretch out your arms and legs and the water is usually not very deep – about 30cm (1ft) is sufficient. You can float naked or wear a bathing suit depending on your preference and the club's house rules. After a flotation session, drink plenty of mineral water to help your body flush out and rehydrate. Then take it easy for a few hours to recuperate.

38 aromatherapy massage

Essential oils have powerful healing properties. Both fennel and juniper are potent detoxifiers and are wonderful for a hangover. Use them in an aromatherapy self-massage.

fennel oil

According to folklore, fennel was believed to offer protection against the evil eye. Today the plant's essential oil is recognized for its effectiveness in counteracting the effects of alcoholic poisoning: it has been used successfully in the treatment and rehabilitation of alcoholics. This may be because fennel is a diuretic and a powerful detoxifier. It also has a calming effect on an upset digestive system and gives speedy relief from nausea and acid indigestion.

juniper oil

When the body needs to detoxify, juniper is ideal. It stimulates the body into throwing off toxic wastes and, like fennel, is a diuretic. Juniper is also good for cleansing and purifying on a mental and emotional level, helping to clear away any negativity picked up during social interaction.

Juniper has a strong smell that is surprisingly pleasant when diluted and used in blends. Its characteristic smoky note combines well with the fresh, aniseed-like aroma of fennel. To treat a hangover, one of the best ways of using the oils is through massage.

Essential oils should never be used directly on the skin but mixed in a suitable carrier base, such as sweet almond oil or an unscented lotion. Add 5 drops of fennel and 3 drops of juniper to 30ml/2 tbsp oil or lotion and mix well. If you wish, you could also add a couple of drops of lemon oil to give it a refreshing, citrus tang. Massage the oil into your thighs, upper back, arms and shoulders using smooth, circling movements.

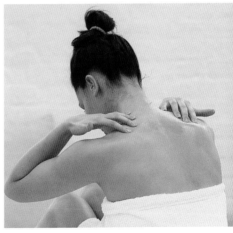

▲ Use essential oils of juniper, fennel and lemon in an aromatherapy massage. It will help with your hangover detox.

39 hangover headache easer

Two of the best essential oils for a hangover headache are lavender and peppermint. When used together they make a formidable combination. You can use them in a balm.

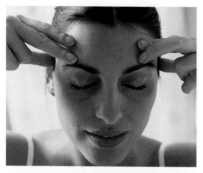

▲ Gently rub a little balm into your temples with your fingertips for headache relief.

The most important constituent of peppermint oil is menthol. When your head is heavy and you can't think straight, the smell of peppermint is like a breath of fresh air that will blow away the cobwebs. Lavender oil also has a refreshing aroma, although its effect is more calming and balancing.

Both peppermint and lavender oils are anti-inflammatory with analgesic (pain-relieving) properties. They are complementary to one another, each enhancing the action of the other. Peppermint is a stimulant and lavender a sedative. This combination of stimulant and sedative is found in many commercial pain-killing

preparations but there is an important difference: essential oils not only kill the pain but they also get to work on its underlying causes. Used correctly, they are also non-toxic.

lavender and peppermint balm

To ease a hangover headache, make up your own lavender and peppermint balm and keep it on standby. Use 3 drops each of lavender and peppermint to every 60ml/4 tbsp unscented base cream. Blend the oils into the cream and keep in a screw-top jar. When you need to use, massage a little into your temples.

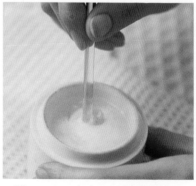

▲ It is easy to make up a headache balm using lavender and peppermint oils.

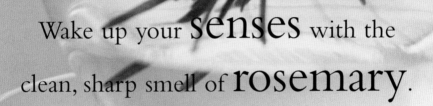

Wake up your senses with the clean, sharp smell of rosemary.

Vaporize a few drops of the essential oil in a burner for an instant hangover cure to leave you refreshed and ready for a new day.

41 relaxing lavender bath

Lavender is one of nature's great cure-all remedies. Its many amazing properties will soon restore you – particularly when combined with a relaxing warm bath.

The association between lavender and bathing goes back a long way. The word lavender is taken from the Latin word *lavare*, meaning 'to wash', possibly because it was used to cleanse wounds, although it also has a long tradition of use in personal bathing. Lavender has a refreshing, sweet scent and is one of the most versatile and popular essential oils. It is an anti-depressant, anti-inflammatory, sedative, mild diuretic and painkiller, with an overall soothing and relaxing effect.

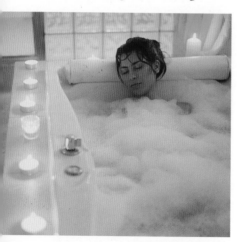

▲ Bathing in a lavender-scented bath should help restore your equilibrium.

However, lavender's most important therapeutic property is that it is balancing: lavender is most useful for bringing body and mind back to a state of equilibrium in which healing can take place.

lavender bath
If this sounds just what you need to help shake off your hangover, then try adding 6-8 drops of lavender oil to a warm bath. Because essential oils do not dissolve in water, you need to swish the water thoroughly to help the oil droplets disperse. If you prefer, you could also mix the oil with 15ml/ 1 tbsp of cream or honey before adding it to the bath. Lie back in the water for at least ten minutes to allow the oil to enter your system and do its work. Taking a lavender bath is an excellent way to help prepare for a good night's sleep as the warm, fragrant water will relax body and mind and help settle an over-stimulated system. If you have very sensitive skin and prefer not to bathe using essential oil, you could tie a bundle of dried lavender under the running taps for a similar effect.

42 citrus spritzer

When you want the world to stop, a fragrant mist of citrus scents will refresh your spirits and give you a boost. It's an instant quick fix that is easy to prepare.

When life has to go on regardless of how you feel, an emergency quick-fix solution is called for.

Without having to eat or drink a single thing, a quick burst of on-the-spot aromatherapy can give you a lift and change your mood. Whether or not you are aware of it, different scents influence the way that you feel. This is because your sense of smell is registered in the area of the brain that is associated with moods, emotions and instinctive responses. Citrus scents are refreshing, tangy and revitalizing. A handy way of using them is in a mist-sprayer.

emergency reviver
For an instant energizer, make a mix containing three distinctive, but complementary, citrus scents: lemon, grapefruit, and bergamot. Bergamot oil is one of the essential ingredients in eau-de-Cologne toilet water and is what gives Earl Grey tea its distinctive scent and flavour. It is uplifting and reviving. The fresh, clean, lively scent of lemon dispels sluggishness and will put you in a better frame of mind, while the tangy,

sweet aroma of grapefruit will also lighten your mood and give you a kick start into action. To make a mist-spray add 150ml/¼ pint/⅔ cup water to a spray bottle (tap water is fine). Then add 6 drops of bergamot and 5 drops each of lemon and grapefruit. Shake the bottle well before you spray to help the oil droplets disperse. Hold the mister about 30cm/1ft away from you and spritz away. Make sure that you do not spray directly onto your eyes or any polished surfaces.

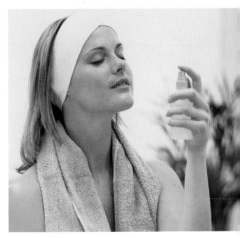

▲ *An aromatic mist of bergamot, lemon and grapefruit is an instant pick-me-up.*

43

camomile compress

When you have a hangover you need to be especially gentle with yourself. Camomile is one of the mildest and most soothing of all the essential oils. Give it a try.

In Ancient Egypt, the camomile plant was dedicated to the sun god, Ra, for its effectiveness in bringing down a fever. Camomile is soothing and anti–inflammatory, which makes it especially useful for dealing with excess heat in the body. Too much alcohol aggravates the body's delicate internal balance and produces an acid, over–heated system. This not only shows up on a physical level but also affects mood and emotions. With a hangover, acid indigestion and sickness is often accompanied by irritability and anxiety and these are all signs that the body is under stress.

Camomile is one of the best remedies for a generally upset system. It is especially effective for digestive disorders, particularly when stomach cramps and diarrhoea are present. On a mental level, it is calming and soothing for all states of anger or agitation. Like lavender, camomile's overall effect is to rebalance the body's energies and restore harmony.

stomach soothing compress

If your hangover is accompanied by griping stomach pains and you feel generally unwell, a camomile compress over your abdomen is a gentle but effective treatment. To make the compress you need a piece of clean cotton cloth and a bowl of hand-hot water. About 300ml/ ½ pint/1¼ cups water should be sufficient. Add 6 drops of camomile to the water and stir well. Soak the cloth in the water, allowing it to absorb the oils. Squeeze it lightly and position it over your abdomen for 10-15 minutes. Lie back and relax.

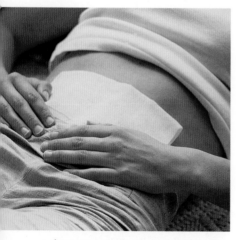

▲ A warm camomile compress over your abdomen can relieve stomach pains.

44 aromatic facial

Frequent excessive drinking is ageing and damaging to your complexion. Give your face a morning-after treat with an aromatic facial – a steam followed by a rich moisturizer.

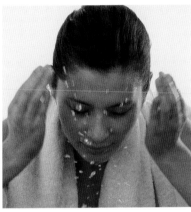

▲ *Splashing your face with water will leave your skin tingly and refreshed.*

You may not be aware of it, but your face will eventually register the telltale signs of all your alcoholic binges. Drinking a lot of alcohol puts pressure on the delicate blood vessels in your face. Constant dilation of these vessels strains the fibrous connective tissue and the vessel walls will eventually collapse, with your skin losing its suppleness and elasticity. Dehydration caused by drinking will also take its toll: your skin will dry out and any facial lines will look more pronounced.

refreshing facial

If this doesn't sound too good, then it's a good idea to minimize the damage by giving your skin an extra nourishing treat after you've been out on the town. An aromatic facial uses essential oils in various ways. A good place to start is with a steam treatment. Put 2-3 drops of geranium oil in a bowl of near-boiling water. Close your eyes and sit in the steam for about five minutes. For a stronger effect, you could also make a 'tent' with a towel draped over your head and the bowl to capture the steam. The steam will open your pores while geranium is cleansing and refreshing for all skin types.

Once your skin feels clean, splash your face with some icy cold spring water to close the pores. By now your skin should feel tingly and be beginning to lose its death-mask appearance. Leave your skin to settle for 15 minutes or so before applying a rich moisturizer. For a nourishing and rejuvenating cream, mix 4 drops of rose and 2 drops of frankincense with 60ml/4 tbsp unscented base cream. Store in a screw-top jar.

Hangovers are heavy on the eyes.

Try the classic

cucumber cure

– lie back with a slice of cucumber

over **each eye** and that nasty

puffy red look should just disappear.

Cucumbers are **cooling and refreshing** and contain

valuable properties that help the eyes.

46 take it easy

Having a hangover is nature's way of saying, 'stop'. Your body needs a chance to rest and recuperate and you have every excuse to stay at home and take it easy.

Admit it, there's a part of you that's secretly glad that you feel so bad. It means no work, no one to tell you what to do, and an excuse to lie back with your feet up. So take the phone off the hook, listen to some relaxing music, graze on snacks and watch television or a video. If you feel up to it, you may even want to read – but nothing too strenuous, perhaps your favourite magazine or that paperback that's been lying around for ages.

rest your over-worked system

Before you start to feel guilty, remember that a hangover puts an enormous strain on your body. You are severely dehydrated and your brain seems to have shrunk to the size of a walnut. Without moving a muscle, your liver and kidneys are working overtime to pump out the poisons, your heart is working extra hard and you are losing valuable nutrients. On top of it all, you didn't sleep well last night. You tried drinking black coffee to sober you up but all that did was keep you awake. When you lay down you felt giddy and had to get up and run to the bathroom. This morning you had to clean it up. It's no wonder you feel so gruesome.

So stop fighting and give in. Keep your fluid intake high, eat something nutritious (if you can) and let nature take its course. The effects of a hangover last about 24 hours so be patient – you'll soon feel better and ready to do it all over again.

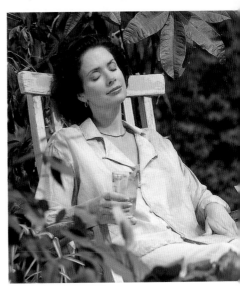

▲ A hangover is the perfect excuse to sit back, relax and put your feet up.

47 pump it out

If you work out regularly you'll find that your hangover recovery time is shortened. Once you're over the very worst of it, you may even feel like taking some exercise.

feel the benefit

Everyone knows that exercise is good for you. It boosts circulation, increases heart rate and builds stamina and strong muscles. It is also one of the best ways of releasing stress. When you are stressed, the body produces extra adrenaline as its fight/flight mechanism gets triggered. When this is not used up, it gets stored in your body as toxic waste. Vigorous exercise (the kind that makes you sweat) helps your body to release toxins, leading to a natural 'high', because it raises your endorphin levels, lifting your spirits and making you feel better. It also builds immunity and helps you recover faster when you do get sick.

know your limitations

Exercising will help you recover from a hangover but only if you work within your 'feel-good' limits. Now is not the time to start working-out with a vengeance if you are not used to it. Take a walk in the fresh air or dig the garden for an hour or so. You could also try cleaning and tidying up the house as that will get your circulation moving without being too taxing. Once you are on the road to recovery, you may feel up to doing something a little more vigorous. Choose an activity that you enjoy, such as going to the gym, power walking, jogging, dancing, cycling or swimming. It will help your body get rid of any lingering toxins and really knock your hangover on its head. Remember to drink plenty of water.

▲ Dancing is fun. It keeps you fit and helps you to get over a hangover faster.

48 mind-bending meditation

One of the good things about meditation is that it can give you a natural lift without any nasty repercussions later. It is also healing for mind, body and soul.

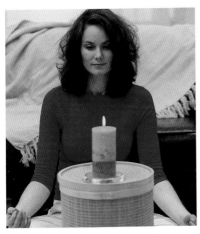

▲ *Meditation helps bring you back into balance and a place of inner calm.*

Studies have shown that the level of relaxation experienced during meditation can be more profound than sleep, which may help to explain why some monks and yogis are able to go without sleep for long periods of time and yet remain serene and calm. Unfortunately this is not the case for most of us. One bad night's sleep and you tend to feel like death warmed up – and that's without the drinking. Add alcohol to the mix and it's no wonder you feel so grim.

The good news is that even ten minutes of meditation can work wonders and minimize the damage. The following meditation uses sound.

humming meditation
Certain sounds send relaxing signals to body and mind. This meditation uses humming which sets up a healing vibration in your body. Sit in a quiet spot where you won't be disturbed and make yourself comfortable. Your spine needs to be as straight as possible, but make sure your back is well supported. Close your eyes and let your breathing settle. As you breathe out let yourself make a humming sound, feeling the vibration of the sound through your body. As you do so, visualize your body being filled with golden yellow light. Keep the humming going for about five minutes, breathing in and humming as you breathe out. You should find that the length of your hums increases as you relax more deeply. When the humming stops, sit quietly for another five minutes continuing to visualize the golden light filling your body. Get up slowly at the end.

49

get intimate

When you and your partner both have the hangover from hell, what better way to commiserate than by getting intimate with one another. It could make you both feel better.

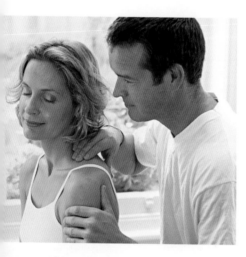

◄ *Touch is one of the best natural therapies of all. Try it with your partner.*

Although sex is probably the last thing on your mind right now, you could start off with a little touch therapy. Touch is an instinctive response to pain and in the right hands is very healing. Hippocrates, the famous physician from Ancient Greece, recommended that every doctor should be experienced in 'rubbing'. This is because the skin is the body's largest sensory organ. Skin contains thousands of receptors that react to external stimuli by transmitting messages through the nervous system to the brain.

sensual healing

Being stroked, rubbed or touched in a sensitive, loving way not only feels good, but also triggers the release of endorphins, your body's natural analgesics or painkillers. It also boosts circulation and helps to oxygenate your blood, improving the flow of vital nutrients through your body. Massage improves lymphatic drainage and stimulates the removal of toxins. It also boosts immunity, eases muscular tension and dissolves energy blocks so that your body's natural healing energies can freely flow.

You don't need to know any special strokes to give your partner a massage, but let your intuition be your guide. Who knows – there's every chance that as you relax and start feeling good together, your sexual desire may start to ignite. So give it a try – for sex is one of the best natural therapies of all. Best of all, you can do it without having to get up – and afterwards you may drift into a peaceful slumber.

50

snooze & sleep

Too much booze affects your sleep. The chances are you didn't get very much last night and have woken up feeling like something that the cat dragged in.

To cure a hangover, take a tip from domestic cats. They spend most of their lives asleep. Anytime, anywhere (so long as it's warm) they snooze their way to dreamland, pictures of utter bliss and relaxation.

disturbed sleep

If only it were that simple. You've spent the whole night tossing and turning, up and down to the bathroom. When you fell asleep, the alcohol in your system drugged your brain and interfered with your body's normal sleep pattern. Critically, you were unable to enter the important REM (rapid eye movement) stage that is associated with dreaming and which is critical to a good night's rest. This lack of refreshing dream sleep is one of the reasons why you feel so irritable, bad-tempered and exhausted, along with just about everything else bad that you can think of.

restorative catnaps

Sleep is one of nature's greatest healers. During sleep your body's cells renew and repair themselves and your brain is able to process information.

Sleep is relaxing and rejuvenating and is really one of the best hangover cures of all. So take plenty of catnaps during the day and have an early night. You'll wake up full of bounce and ready to face the world. If you have trouble dropping off, a warm milky drink flavoured with nutmeg can help.

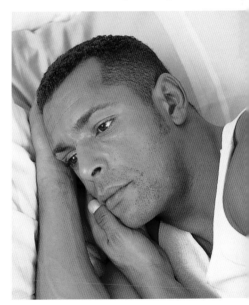

▲ Give in to tiredness and take a nap. Sleep is probably the simplest, and yet greatest, healer of them all.

index

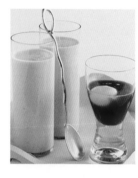

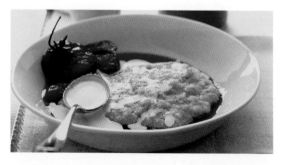

index

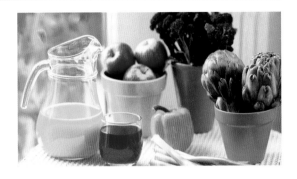

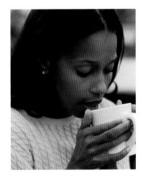

This edition is published by Lorenz Books, an imprint of Anness Publishing Ltd,
Blaby Road, Wigston, Leicestershire LE18 4SE; info@anness.com

www.lorenzbooks.com; www.annesspublishing.com

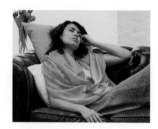

If you like the images in this book and would like to investigate using them for
publishing, promotions or advertising, please visit our website
www.practicalpictures.com for more information.

Publisher: Joanna Lorenz
Managing editor: Helen Sudell
Editor: Melanie Halton
Designer: Ian Sandom
Photography: Michelle Garrett, Christine Hanscomb, Don Last,
Liz McAulay, and Fiona Pragoff.
Production controller: Steve Lang

PUBLISHER'S NOTE
The reader should not regard the recommendations, ideas and techniques expressed and
described in this book as substitutes for the advice of a qualified medical practitioner or
other qualified professional. Any use to which the recommendations, ideas and
techniques are put is at the reader's sole discretion and risk.

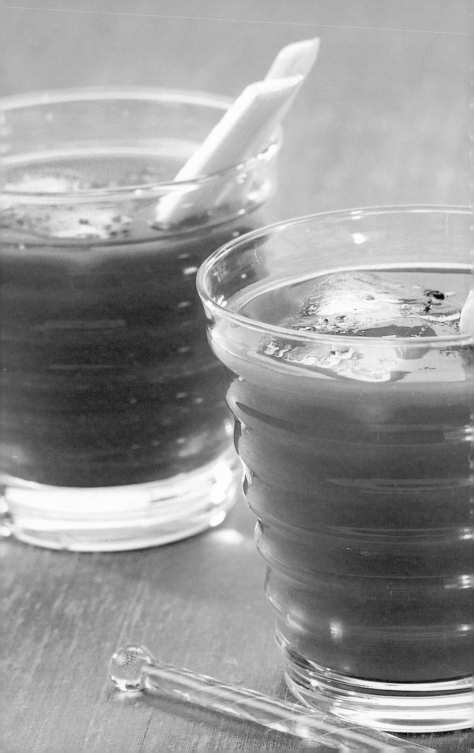